Leaky Gut Syndrome STOP!

A Complete Guide To Leaky Gut Syndrome Causes, Symptoms, Treatments & A Holistic System To Eliminate LGS Naturally & Permanently

Melanie J. Smith
Copyright© 2014 by Melanie J. Smith

Leaky Gut Syndrome STOP!

Publisher: Enlightened Publishing

ISBN-13: 978-1499768398

ISBN-10: 1499768397

Disclaimer

The Publisher has strived to be as accurate and complete as possible in the creation of this book. While all attempts have been made to verify information provided in this publication, the Publisher assumes no responsibility for errors, omissions, or contrary interpretation of the subject matter herein. Any perceived slights of specific persons, peoples, or organizations are unintentional.

This book is not intended for use as a source of legal, business, accounting or financial advice. All readers are advised to seek services of competent professionals in the legal, business, accounting, and finance fields.

The information in this book is not intended or implied to be a substitute for professional medical advice, diagnosis or treatment. All content contained in this book is for general information purposes only. Always consult your healthcare provider before carrying on any health program.

Table of Contents

Introduction

Leaky gut syndrome is a condition in which the gut passes things it shouldn't pass into the bloodstream. In Chapter 1, we will talk a close look at leaky gut syndrome, what it does and why it is so harmful to your body. But first, let's have a crash course on our digestive system.

Ideally, food is digested as it travels from mouth to anus. Digestion is the process of breaking down food into smaller molecules so they can easily pass through the intestinal wall into the bloodstream around the intestine. Without digestion, food would pass through the intestines unchanged and we would starve.

The gastrointestinal tract is used each and every day by the average person. Food is first chewed and partially digested by enzymes in the saliva. The food is swallowed in boluses or "bites" of food that are chewed significantly so they can have a bigger surface area to be acted upon by the stomach later. The oral cavity contains the enzymes called *lingual lipase*, which initiates lipid digestion, *amylase*, which aids carbohydrate digestion, *mucin*, which lubricates the food and *lysozyme*, which helps sanitize food.

The food then travels down the esophagus and lands in the acidic environment of the stomach. The esophagus is the long tube extending from the back of the throat or pharynx to the stomach. It pushes food boluses down into the stomach using involuntary wave movements that are called peristalsis. This allows the passage of food even against gravity.

Once the food empties into the stomach, it is partially digested by stomach acids, which denature protein and break down carbohydrates into smaller components, creating a substance called "chyme". The stomach contains high concentrations of hydrochloric acid which activates pepsinogen into *pepsin*, which breaks down protein molecules into amino acids and small polypeptide fragments. *Intrinsic factor* is also produced by the parietal cells of the stomach that is important in the absorption of vitamin B12.

Both mucin and stomach acid are active in killing off dangerous bacteria within the stomach so they don't pass through the stomach and into the intestines. The hormone *gastrin* is produced by the G cells within the stomach. It is an enzyme and hormone that enters the bloodstream to stimulate the production of hydrochloric acid within the stomach. It is turned on when the stomach is distended with food.

The food then leaves the stomach and travels to the duodenum. There, pancreatic enzymes are secreted through the Ampulla of Vater, an opening in the duodenum that allows the passage of both bile and pancreatic enzymes into the duodenum.

The pancreas produces bicarbonate that neutralizes the acidic contents of the chyme from the stomach so the enzymes of the pancreas can begin to work under a less acidic environment. The acinar cells of the pancreas produce inactive pancreatic enzymes that are activated in the environment of the small intestines.

Pancreatic juices contain *trypsinogen*, which breaks down proteins into amino acids, *chymotrypsinogen*, which also breaks down proteins into amino acids, *carboxypeptidase*, which removes the terminal amino acid group from the end of a protein and *pancreatic lipase*, an enzyme that turns triglycerides in food into glycerol and fatty acids. Miscellaneous enzymes produced in the pancreas are *elastases, cholesterol esterase, phospholipase* and *pancreatic lipase*. There are also enzymes that break down DNA and RNA of cells and *pancreatic amylase*, which breaks down carbohydrates. What it can't do is break down cellulose, which becomes a fibrous substance in our waste products.

The duodenum secretes hormones and proteins that regulate digestion. These include *secretin, cholecystokinin* or CCK, which is released in response to high protein or fat content in the chyme. CCK causes the gallbladder to contract so that bile can be squeezed into the duodenum. Bile works to break down fats into fatty acids.

In the small intestine, consisting of the duodenum, jejunum and ileum, digestion and absorption occur equally. Food is digested in the duodenum and is primarily absorbed in the jejunum. It is the longest section of the small intestine and contains millions of villi that promote absorption of nutrients. The ileum is the last portion of the small intestines. It absorbs bile for re-use and absorbs vitamin B12, with the help of intrinsic factor produced in the stomach.

Along the lining of the small intestines, there are many different enzymes referred to as "brush border enzymes". They are enzymes that further digest the food particles so that they can be absorbed. They include several enzymes called *sucrase*, *lactase*, *maltase* and other *disaccharidases*.

The function of the large intestine or colon is to hold feces, which are the waste products of digestion. Some of the water and electrolytes within the colon are absorbed back into the bloodstream so that stool is thicker than the material passed through it by the small intestines. There are bacteria in the large intestines such as Bacteroides species, Lactobacillus species, E. coli and Klebsiella that act to further digest waste products.

Solid waste is then passed through the rectum and anus in a bowel movement. This completes what is essentially a normal digestive process. But what happens when the digestive process goes wrong and when the wrong things get absorbed into the small intestine? Well, let's read on to find that out.

Chapter 1: Leaky Gut Syndrome – What Is It?

Leaky gut syndrome is a condition where the bowel lining is damaged in some way causing an increase in the ability of molecules larger than simple carbohydrates, fatty acids, amino acids and vitamins to enter the bloodstream. It can be a result eating a poor diet, parasitic organisms, food that is undigested, bacteria, or certain medications.

The idea behind leaky gut syndrome is that the organisms or undigested food is recognized by the body as being foreign and the body makes antibodies to the substance, creating an unwanted immune response. In fact, some doctors believe that leaky gut syndrome or LGS can contribute to many different diseases as well as chronic complaints other doctors can't figure out.

The pathology that explains leaky gut syndrome is an inflammation or irritation of the lining of the small intestines due to reasons explained above. This allows toxic agents from the food or from bacteria to enter the bloodstream rather than pass through to the colon in a process known as increased *intestinal permeability*. In layman's terms, this means the gut is leaky and allows the passage of things it shouldn't pass through to the bloodstream.

Because leaky gut is believed to play a role in the immune system, it is believed to cause several different conditions, such as hives, eczema of the skin, asthma (which affects the lungs), rheumatoid arthritis and other autoimmune joint diseases, fibromyalgia, chronic sinus infections, food allergies, PMS, fibroids in the breast and uterus and chronic fatigue syndrome. Childhood immune deficiencies seem also to be related to leaky gut syndrome.

What can cause this condition? We will discuss the causes more in details in Chapter 3. Not all causes of leaky gut syndrome have been determined; however, antibiotic use is believed to be one way of destroying the lining of the small bowel. While antibiotics kill dangerous bacteria, they also have a way of destroying healthy and beneficial bacteria in both the small and large intestine. We need these bacteria for proper digestion of food and to create an environment where food is digested completely.

Nonsteroidal anti-inflammatory medication has been implicated in leaky gut syndrome. These include NSAIDS like ibuprofen, naproxen and rofecoxib, marketed as Motrin®, Advil®, Aleve® and Vioxx®. These agents are known to damage the lining of the stomach and are believed to damage the lining of the small intestines as well.

Bacteria contain enzymes of their own that further break down waste products, bile, cellular debris, bad bacteria, and toxins from viruses and bacteria that would otherwise get absorbed and cause a negative immune response. When these bacteria are gotten rid of by antibiotics, it paves the way for either few bacteria or bad bacteria and fungi to take the place of the beneficial bacteria, leading to a toxic environment in the small and large intestines.

If the bile is not digested properly, it can damage the lining of the large bowel. Normally, it is an extremely beneficial substance, digesting fats into fatty acids, acting as a lubricant within the small intestines and detoxifying toxins that build up in the liver. In the large bowel, however, it is unwanted and needs the presence of beneficial bacteria to render it non-toxic. Some believe that, in the absence of beneficial bacteria, the caustic bile can irritate the lining of the large bowel, leading to colon cancer.

The beneficial colonic bacteria are also responsible for the metabolism of hormones such as estrogen, which are passed through the liver into the small intestines in the bile. If the bacteria are unavailable to digest estrogen, for example, and if the small intestine is leaky, the estrogen gets reabsorbed within the body, leading to estrogen excess. This may, in turn, cause symptoms of PMS, uterine fibroids and estrogen-responsive tumors of the breast or uterus.

Without beneficial bacteria, the colon and small intestine can be overrun with *Candida*, a type of yeast, and other fungi. This is what is believed to be the main trigger behind getting a leaky gut. The normal lining of the gut has tight connections between the cells so that absorption is basically well controlled and only small molecules can get through. Candida secretes a type of aldehyde that shrinks the lining cells of the intestinal wall so that there is a bigger opening for larger molecules and bacteria to pass between the cells.

Besides altering the physical barrier in the intestinal wall, Candida affects the "chemical barrier" of the intestinal lining. This chemical barrier is contained within the mucus of the small intestines and protects the body from toxins that might pass through the intestinal wall. It consists of immune molecules that can recognize and destroy toxic agents. Without the physical barrier, the immune barrier becomes overwhelmed and allows the passage of toxic agents into the body.

There were once some theories which indicated that Candida entered the bloodstream itself, landing in the brain or other body cells. The truth of the matter is that, unless a person has HIV or AIDS, the Candida is sought after in the bloodstream and is destroyed by our immune system.

Rather than do damage by entering the bloodstream itself, it allows toxic agents and undigested food particles to enter the blood. The body will see some of these food particles as foreign bodies and will want to make antibodies against the "foreigners". This leads to an inflammatory immune response and food allergies that persist anytime the offending food is ingested. The food allergies remain, even after the problem with the yeast is long over with.

Common food allergies include allergies to eggs, dairy products and grains containing gluten, such as wheat, rye, and oats, nuts, corn, and soybeans. Allergies to things like rice, fruits, vegetables or meat are much less common.

A true allergic reaction involves the release of histamine, which causes hives and stomach discomfort. An ordinary sensitivity to food products yields gassiness, abdominal discomfort, nausea and diarrhea but it does not necessarily mean you have a food allergy. You need to have allergy testing to see what it is you are allergic to.

When toxins are allowed into the body, you can get inflammation of tissues, deposition of toxic substances, swollen lymph glands, muscle and body aches, joint pain, "brain fog" and a reduction in the energy produced by the body. This is when diseases like chronic arthritis, fibromyalgia, cancer and other gene mutations can occur within the body. The body stresses itself out trying to get rid of undigested food and toxins. In addition, the liver becomes stressed trying to deactivate toxins. Ultimately liver damage can occur.

So how does this all work? The Candida results in leaky intestinal membranes and the immune system is activated in response to toxins and partially digested foods entering the body. While some of the toxins aren't inactivated by the intestinal immune system and enter the body, lymphatic system and the liver become overwhelmed. The immune system is overwhelmed overall so that it can't fight off opportunistic infections that enter the body through the GI tract or through other sources. Eventually the function of the adrenal gland is diminished so that your cortisol levels decrease and you become exhausted and unable to function well.

Chapter 2: What Leaky Gut Syndrome Can Do To Your Body?

Leaky gut syndrome can affect many areas of the body. When the gut is leaky, food molecules, hormones and toxins can enter the body and can overload the immune system that is attempting to fight off the offending particles. This leads to a number of conditions and diseases.

Autoimmune Conditions

Leaky gut syndrome can cause multiple problems, including autoimmune diseases. Autoimmune diseases are those diseases in which the body's immune system attacks its own tissues. The gut, being leaky, can allow the passage of particles that can trick the immune system into thinking it is part of your own body. The end result is that, even without the further passage of particles, the immune system is turned on to fighting your tissues.

Which diseases are more likely to result from leaky gut syndrome due to autoimmune mechanisms? Let's take a look:

- **Systemic lupus erythematosus (SLE)**: This an autoimmune disease in which multiple connective tissue areas are inflamed, resulting in sore joints, kidney disease, heart problems, nervous system disease, liver disease, lung problems, skin diseases and diseases of the blood vessels.

- **Alopecia areata**: This is a disease where there are bald patches or a completely bald scalp from immune antibodies attached to the hair follicles that causes the hair to fall out.

- **Rheumatoid arthritis**: This is a disease where antibodies attack the connective tissue of the joints themselves so that there is joint inflammation, destruction, and deformity of the joints.

- **Polymyalgia rheumatica**: This is a disease where the muscles are affected by antibodies. Most people with the disease have severe stiffness and pain in the neck, shoulders and hips.

- **Multiple sclerosis**: This is a disease where the myelin surrounding the nerves has been destroyed so that the nerves no longer function appropriately and multiple nerve injuries occur.

- **Chronic fatigue syndrome**: While no one knows the exact cause of chronic fatigue syndrome, it may be due to an as yet unknown autoimmune disease that makes a person extremely exhausted and unable to function.

- **Sjogren's syndrome**: This is an autoimmune connective tissue disease that causes dry eyes, dry mouth, and joint aches and pains.

- **Vitiligo**: This is an autoimmune disease in which the skin's melanin is attacked by the body's own immune system, resulting in patches of pure white skin interposed between patches of normal skin.

- **Hashimoto's thyroiditis**: This is a thyroid disease in which there are antibodies against part of the thyroid gland and there is evidence of thyroid dysfunction in most cases.

- **Vasculitis**: This is when the immune system attacks the vascular structures of the body. The end result is bruising, muscle aches and circulation difficulties, especially in the extremities.

- **Crohn's disease**: This is a condition involving any part of the gastrointestinal tract. The GI tract is inflamed and irritated, leading to diarrhea, abdominal pain and possible colon cancer.

- **Ulcerative colitis**: This is a syndrome with much of the same symptoms as Crohn's disease but involves an inflammation of just the colon. Abdominal pain and diarrhea, often bloody, are common.

- **Type I diabetes**: This is an autoimmune disease that affects the islet cells of the pancreas. These cells are destroyed by the immune system and can no longer make insulin to handle the sugar load in the body.

- **Raynaud's disease**: This is a condition in which the hands especially are very cold, even when the rest of the body is warm enough.

So how does leaky gut syndrome cause autoimmune diseases? When the gut is leaky due to a widening of the junctions between the cells of the lining of the GI tract, molecules of food, toxins and other particles get in the bloodstream. The unwanted proteins trigger antibodies to be made against them.

Some proteins strongly resemble receptors on the body's tissue cells. Exactly which tissues are affected varies from protein to protein. The receptors are like a lock on a door. The key to the door is the antibody against the absorbed protein that also happens to fit the receptor "lock". The antibiotic key fits the receptor lock and destroys or inflames the cell. This is what causes an autoimmune disease.

Cells can have antigenic properties that are similar to certain bacteria, parasites, Candida (yeast) or other fungi. These can get into the bloodstream from the intestinal tract and can lead to the same autoimmune diseases that small proteins can. It all depends on the antigenic (receptor) status of the organisms and of the body's tissues.

Food Allergies

In a normal gut, food is broken down into its component parts before getting absorbed. For example, fats are broken down into fatty acids, proteins are broken down into amino acids and complex sugars are broken down into simple sugars. When this process does not happen and larger peptides, sugars and fat substances are allowed to pass through, some of the antigenic properties of the foods they came from are allowed to be exposed to the bloodstream. The end result is food allergies to varying types of food. Common food allergies in leaky gut syndrome include those to:

- Wheat
- Milk
- Eggs
- Corn
- Soy
- Yeast
- Beef
- Legumes, including nuts

- Citrus fruits
- Potatoes
- Tomatoes

What types of food allergies can develop when one has leaky gut syndrome and has food particles (however small) entering the bloodstream and causing an immune response? The food particle becomes the antigen or "allergen" and the antibodies and immune cells react against the allergen:

- **Type I Hypersensitivity**: This is when B lymphocytes (a type of white blood cell) make antibodies to the agent that is believed to be the threat. Antibodies attach to the foreign agent and help the other white blood cells attack and destroy the allergen. This is the most common type of hypersensitivity/allergic reaction. Responses include anaphylaxis and death.

- **IgE-mediated Reactions**: This is when IgE (a type of antibody) binds to mast cells and basophils, making the mast cells active. They then release chemical mediators, including histamine, which makes an allergic reaction. Responses include urticaria or hives, itchy eyes, runny nose, diarrhea, wheezing, nausea and vomiting. Skin reactions such as eczema can occur.

- **Type II Hypersensitivity Reaction**: This is an immune response in which the allergen is already attached to the patient's own tissue. These allergens usually come from an outside source that is ingested by the body. The body uses IgG or IgM antibodies and triggers an attack on the cells themselves. Examples of this type of allergic reaction include autoimmune hemolytic anemia, pernicious anemia and transfusion reactions.

- **Type III Hypersensitivity Reaction**: This involves immune complexes that are soluble in blood (allergen plus antibody together) that become deposited is various places in the body, particularly the joints, kidneys and skin. The body forms an attack against these areas of the body in conditions such as rheumatoid arthritis and systemic lupus erythematosus. The immune complexes plus the surrounding tissue is destroyed, leading to tissue damage.

- **Type IV Hypersensitivity Reaction**: This is also known as T-cell mediated hypersensitivity and is not mediated by antibodies. T-lymphocytes can attack and kill off certain antigens without the need for antibodies. The inflammation seen in the intestinal lining in leaky gut syndrome is believed to be T-cell mediated. Other examples include diabetes mellitus and contact dermatitis. It takes up to 72 hours to get a reaction when exposed to a type IV hypersensitivity allergen.

Many food allergies in leaky gut syndrome are directly related to IgE mediated hypersensitivity reactions. The reactions tend to be relatively immediate and can lead to immediate swelling of the body, urticaria, a drop in blood pressure, asthmatic symptoms, and anaphylaxis.

Increasingly, there are delayed reactions to foods as is sometimes seen in leaky gut syndrome. As it takes several hours or days to exhibit allergic reactions to the allergen, it may be hard to know which food is causing the re-action. Symptoms can be vague and can involve an overall feeling of malaise and fatigue rather than classical allergic symptoms.

Hormonal Effects

Hormones like estrogen can get through the loose junctions between the cells of the lining of the intestinal tract, leading to excess estrogen in the system. Too much estrogen in females can lead to premenstrual syndrome, polyps or fibroids on the uterus, cervical dysplasia, breast tenderness, fibrocystic breast disease, and breast or colon cancer. Estrogen binds to estrogen receptors on female-related body parts such as the uterus, cervix and breasts and causes symptoms of estrogen overload.

In men, estrogen dominance can lead to poor sexual drive and impotence. In severe cases, adrenal exhaustion can occur in both men and women. When the adrenal gland gives out, you won't have enough cortisol and your blood pressure will be uncomfortably low, you'll feel ill, you will lose weight and you will have the possibility of fainting spells.

Other signs of estrogen dominance include evidence of thyroid dysfunction, depression, anxiety, agitation, dry eyes, menstrual cycles that are too close together, endometriosis, hair loss, low blood sugar, foggy thinking, fatigue, gallstones, increased stroke risk, irritability, memory loss, lack of sleep, mood swings, polycystic ovarian syndrome, bone loss before menopause, prostate cancer in men, increased water retention and a deficiencies of magnesium and zinc.

Chronic Fatigue Syndrome

Chronic fatigue syndrome is now known as myalgic encephalomyelitis. It is believed to be an autoimmune disease caused by absorption of viral particles which lead to an immune response and symptoms of myalgias and fatigue. The inflamed gut is also deficient in IgA antibodies, which are the first line of defense in the gut to viral and bacterial microbes. When the immune system gives out on the person, viruses pass through and give rise to chronic fatigue syndrome.

Other common symptoms of chronic fatigue syndrome are confusion, brain fog, memory impairment, and facial swelling when exposed to an irritant. The secondary magnesium, zinc, calcium, and copper deficiency can cause hair loss, elevated blood cholesterol, osteoarthritis and osteoporosis.

Urticaria

Urticaria is also called "hives" and is a direct response to histamine release from mast cells, which are part of the cells of the immune system. When histamine is released in great amounts, there is excessive itching, a red bumpy rash and low blood pressure. The skin itself turns red from histamine release. This happens when IgE senses the presence of an allergen or foreign substance and turns on mast cells, which release histamine.

Normally, this would be part of a typical reaction to a normal pathogen. Unfortunately, in leaky gut syndrome, the histamine is released because of molecules and toxins that have no place being in the bloodstream in the first place. In severe cases, anaphylaxis and death can occur.

Chapter 3: Causes of Leaky Gut Syndrome

Leaky gut syndrome can happen to just about anyone under the right circumstances. Anything that damages the cells of the small intestine so that they shrink and become leaky between the cells will cause an increase in the permeability of the small bowel and the passage of larger particles through the membrane and into the blood stream. There are many things that can cause leaky gut syndrome or can make it worse in those who already have the disease. Let's look at some of the causes and what you can do to prevent the disease from occurring.

Medications

- Antibiotics can cause leaky gut syndrome by ridding the small intestine of normal, beneficial bacteria so that "bad" or pathogenic bacteria can take their place. Later on, we'll talk about how you can use probiotics to better your chances of not getting leaky gut syndrome from antibiotics you can't always avoid taking.

- Nonsteroidal anti-inflammatory medications or NSAIDS are known to irritate and erode the intestinal and stomach surfaces. These include medications such as ibuprofen, aspirin, and naproxen. If you have to take something for pain, take acetaminophen or Tylenol®, which is not an NSAID.

- Birth control pills not only contain excessive estrogen which can get into the system and cause estrogen dominance, it can cause leaky gut syndrome and can result in other symptoms.

- Steroids like prednisone are common causes of leaky gut syndrome because they are known to irritate the lining of the intestinal tract, causing erosions of the esophagus, stomach and intestinal tract. This medication should be taken with food in order to minimize the threat of leaky gut syndrome.

- Chemotherapy medications can be extremely irritating to the lining of the intestinal tract, making the small intestinal cells leakier as a result.

- Antacids can decrease the pH of the stomach, which should be high enough to kill pathogens and to begin the process of digestion. When antacids are used, pathogens can get through to the small intestine and can colonize it. In addition, partially or undigested food particles can travel to the small intestine and are more likely to be taken up in their partially digested form by the leaky gut.

Dietary Patterns

Your diet plays a big role in your getting leaky gut syndrome. If you eat a diet which is high in refined flour, simple and refined sugars, highly processed foods and foods containing chemical additives such as artificial flavors and colors can cause leaky gut syndrome.

Drinks like alcohol, including wine and beer, sodas and caffeinated beverages (or chocolate) can be toxic to the system because they aren't natural substances. Because they aren't natural, they overload the liver that is trying to break down these toxic substances and the immune system becomes overloaded by having to fight off these foreigners. In addition, they can irritate the GI tract lining so that the intestines become leaky.

The Role of Microorganisms

When you consume food, you are also eating bacteria in the food, various parasites, and mycotoxins that are able to damage the lining of the intestinal tract and produce leaky gut syndrome. They also product toxic waste products, gas and other chemicals the body doesn't like.

When these toxic byproducts damage the intestinal lining and pass into the bloodstream, the immune system is touched off and make free radicals that not only attempt to destroy the toxic substance but attack cells and create DNA damage in cells. Free radicals are dangerous the body in high amounts and can damage the lining of the intestinal wall.

Nutritional Deficiency

You need zinc and vitamin B6 in your diet to make the hydrochloric acid that makes the stomach do its job in partially digesting food. These nutrients are also necessary to make the lining of the intestinal tract intact. In addition, vitamin A is necessary for the building of mucosal linings of the intestinal tract. The most important amino acid for intestinal repair is l-glutamine, which repair intestinal linings that are damaged.

Diseases that Cause Leaky Gut

Certain diseases cause an increased permeability of the intestinal tract, such as celiac disease, Crohn's colitis, pancreatitis and HIV/AIDS. HIV causes intestinal permeability because of the strong medications used to manage the condition. Candidiasis or an excess of yeast in the intestinal tract can also lead to leaky gut syndrome and the passage of unhealthy food particles and toxins into the bloodstream.

Those who have certain cancers of the GI tract can have increased permeability of the membranes of the small intestines. Food allergies cause an immune response to build up all along the intestinal tract. The resulting inflammation can cause the intestinal lining to become leaky. Finally, if the liver is overwhelmed or damaged in some way, it can't rid the body of toxins and these toxins feed back onto the intestinal tract and cause a leaky gut. The liver also affects the amount of bile necessary for fat digestion and a lack of bile means intestinal fat remains in the bowels, irritating the bowel.

Lifestyle Factors

If you have a lifestyle that is high in stress, the body suffers from a reduced amount of blood flow to the bowels. This also increases the number and amount of damaging free radicals in the blood.

Nicotine and its related toxins can irritate the lining of the stomach and intestines. Anything that irritates the intestinal lining can contribute to a person getting leaky gut syndrome.

Mechanism of Action

How can all these different agents cause leaky gut syndrome? Notice how some things, like Crohn's disease are both a cause and effect of leaky gut syndrome. This is because diseases and conditions like Crohn's disease can have a self-perpetuating effect on leaky gut syndrome. They both cause the disease and perpetuate it because of an abnormal immune syndrome.

The gut is ideally supposed to let in healthy nutrients while keeping out toxic agents from getting into the bloodstream. It does so by having just the right permeability so that small fatty acids, sugars, amino acids and vitamins, which are not immunogenic, get through the junctions between cells. Certain factors shrink the intestinal cells and increase the space between them. Other factors or conditions increase the space between the cells without altering the cell size.

When the cell junctions increase in size, bacterial fragments, toxins, bacteria and macromolecules (larger molecules) can enter the bloodstream affecting both the immune system and the liver.

How does leaky gut syndrome affect the liver? The liver is responsible for detoxifying the bloodstream and sending toxic molecules from the bloodstream into the bile where they are excreted from the body. Everything that is absorbed by the small intestine goes first to the liver in what's known as enterohepatic circulation. The liver can normally tolerate the load of toxic substances sent to it; however, when too many toxic substances enter the bloodstream and go to the liver, the liver becomes overwhelmed.

In the liver, the cytochrome P450 system is the first phase of detoxification. It is responsible for converting certain free radical molecules to safer molecules and is responsible for making carcinogenic agents less carcinogenic. All of this happens in the liver's Kupffer cells that offer a two stage detoxification process. The second stage involves taking the free radical molecules and carcinogenic agents and metabolizing them through conjugation (connection) with glutathione, glycine, sulfate or glucuronide. These conjugated agents are completely safe and are secreted through the biliary system and out into the bowels.

Sometimes the capacity of the phase 2 part of this detoxification process becomes depleted and exhausted, resulting in an overflow of carcinogenic agents and free radicals within the liver. This causes damage to the liver and overflow of these agents into the bloodstream where they damage cells and create problems like cellular apoptosis (cell death) and cancerous cells. The liver can be further challenged by the addition of acetaminophen, caffeine or aspirin, making the liver more overwhelmed than before.

The GI tract is actually the biggest immune organ within the body. It needs to be so because there are many toxic and immune-producing organisms and molecules the GI tract comes in contact with. It is an interface between the outside of our bodies and the inside of our bodies. When the junctions between the cells of the intestinal tract are increased, too many bacteria, bacterial fragments and toxic molecules get into the body, triggering an immune response. Antibodies to these substances form and this turns on the immune effects within the body.

When the immune system is overtaxed by macromolecules and bacteria/bacterial fragments, four things can happen:

- The nutrients and reserves of the immune system are depleted.

- Autoimmune reactions can happen by having an immune complex be too close to the antigenic properties of a normal bodily tissue, such as the joints, connective tissue, nerves, lung and skin.

- The antigenic load to the body becomes too large for too long, leading to a "hyperimmune state" and immune overload.

- The antigen and antibody complex can irritate and inflame the wall of the gut so that the gut feeds back on itself and becomes even more leaky. This is a self-perpetuating cycle.

What this means is that the leaky gut syndrome affects not only the gut but the liver function and immune system as well. Patients begin to get an active, clinical disease or at least a decrease in overall wellness.

How is leaky gut syndrome a self-perpetuating cycle? It is so in several different ways:

- When a person develops a food allergy from a case of leaky gut syndrome, the food causes an allergic reaction in the gut that further increases gut permeability. This means more partially-digested food particles are allowed to pass through the leaky GI junctions. Stopping the offending food is the only way to break the cycle.

- Leaky gut produces malabsorption so there is a lack of proper nutrients getting to the small intestinal cells. These cells become atrophic (shrink) and this makes leaky gut syndrome even worse. Good nutrition to the GI tract can help improve the situation.

- The disordered intestinal bacterial milieu both causes leaky gut syndrome and is perpetuates the syndrome. The bacteria, which are harmful to the gut, cause the gut to become leaky. Then bacterial fragments and bacteria can pass through the GI tract, triggering an immune response. The antigen-antibody immune response then feeds back and causes the GI tract to become more inflamed and increasingly leaky. The best way to manage this is to clear out the offending bacteria and return the bacterial milieu to normal.

- The leaky gut is related to an imbalance in the liver's ability to detoxify danger-ous molecules and the bile becomes overflowing with free radicals. These free radicals are discharged into the in-testinal tract where they can worsen the intestinal tract's permeability. The only treatment is to stop whatever it is that is causing the leaky gut syndrome in the first place.

Leaky gut is caused by many different things, some of which have the added disad-vantage of feeding back on the GI tract, creat-ing a self-perpetuating cycle. Many people are in this cycle and don't know that their symp-toms are from leaky gut syndrome. As noted in the previous chapter, there are many differ-ent symptoms of leaky gut syndrome and, even when you suspect you have the disease, it is difficult to know what the offending agent is.

For this reason, you need to be aware of the various causes of leaky gut syndrome and know which causes have a self-perpetuating feature. Those that do are especially dangerous because it takes an action on your part to get rid of the disease. Even those causes that are not self-perpetuating can be difficult to pinpoint and subsequently get rid of.

As you have probably already discovered, leaky gut syndrome is just one small part of the overall problem. When offending agents cause an increase in the permeability of the GI tract, it affects the liver, the immune system and places like the joints, connective tissue, nerves, uterus, breasts, adrenal glands and other body parts. Exactly what symptoms you have depends on the causative factors and on the often unpredictable nature of what can enter the blood stream from a leaky gut.

You want to avoid as many of the causative factors of leaky gut syndrome as possible so your gut, immune system, liver and other organs remain optimally functioning and healthy.

Chapter 4: Diagnosis of Leaky Gut Syndrome

Leaky gut syndrome can be tested for although there are only a few laboratories that test for the disease. You need a doctor's order to have the tests done but if your doctor is open-minded about the possibility of disease, he or she will happily order the necessary tests for you. We'll talk about the places you can send samples to in order to check for leaky gut syndrome at the end of this chapter.

What Conditions Signal the Need for Testing?

If you have any one of the following diseases, you should consider the possibility that you might have leaky gut syndrome and should seek medical evaluation and testing:

- Arthritis, especially if it is related to an autoimmune disease like rheumatoid arthritis

- Allergies, particularly if you have food allergies

- Depression, including symptoms of malaise and fatigue with low energy and low mood

- Eczema, which is an allergic skin disease affecting primarily the face and the inner aspects of the elbows or behind the knees

- Hives, which are intensely itchy red bumps on the skin caused by an allergic reaction and histamine release

- Psoriasis, which is an autoimmune condition affecting the outer aspects of the elbows and outer aspects of the knees primarily

- Chronic fatigue syndrome or myalgic encephalomyelitis is a condition where you have constant malaise, fatigue and feelings of being run down and achy.

- Fibromyalgia, which is chronic disease of musculoskeletal pain and aching

Once you come to realize that leaky gut syndrome is behind one of the above conditions, you'll have a better time determining how to treat it. Treat the underlying condition and the more obvious disease disappears without any added treatment. There are other conditions that are less common which are contributcd to by having lcaky gut syndromc. See Chapter 2 and, if you have any of those diseases, talk to your doctor about the possibility of leaky gut syndrome.

As mentioned, there are tests for leaky gut syndrome that can be performed to show whether or not you have the disease. Let's take a look at some of these important tests:

- **Polyethylene Glycol Test or PEG Test.** This is perhaps the most commonly performed test for leaky gut syndrome. In the test, the test individual is provided with a solution of lactulose and mannitol. Lactulose is an indigestible, disaccharide sugar under normal circumstances and mannitol is a monosaccharide alcoholic sugar related to sorbitol. The person consumes the concoction and collects their urine for six hours post-ingestion. Neither sugar is metabolized by the body; mannitol is easily absorbed while lactulose is only partially absorbed due to its large nature. If there are high levels of both mannitol and lactulose in the subject's urine then leaky gut syndrome is assumed to exist. If the levels of both sugars are low, then one must assume a diagnosis of malabsorption. If the levels of mannitol are high and the levels of lactulose are low, the person is to be considered to have normal digestion.

- **Digestive Stool Analysis.** This is a direct evaluation of the stool, which contains the products of all things left undigested in the bowels. It looks at the absorption of proteins, fats, carbohydrates and nutrients from the food. It also looks for the presence of Candida yeast species and it cultures the stool for the most prevalent bacteria. If dysbiosis exists, unhealthy pathogenic bacteria will be prominent in the culture. In addition, the presence of parasites in the stool can indicate the presence of leaky gut syndrome.

- **Candida Testing.** The stool can be cultured for Candidiasis and the doctor can check for levels of the IgA, IgM and IgG antibodies against Candida species. This would indicate that Candida has gotten into the bloodstream at one point and has activated an antibody response. A positive IgG level indicates a chronic or past Candida exposure, while a positive IgM level means there is an acute or active infection going on. IgA antibodies are surface antibodies activated in places like the sinus tract, the oral mucosa and the GI tract.

- **Allergy Testing (also called Intolerance or Sensitivity Testing).** The doctor can do one of several tests including a skin prick or scratch test in which fluid is dropped in a drop-by-drop fashion onto the skin and the skin is scratched, allowing for some of the solution to get into the bloodstream. If you're allergic to the substance, then a small (or large) red bump will appear where the scratch was. It is usually done on the forearm, the back or the upper arm, depending on how many scratch tests will be needed. The doctor looks especially for things like food allergies and allergies to other substances ingested by the body.

Another allergy test is the blood RAST test also called the radioallergosorbent test. This exposes the body to various allergens and measures the amount of IgE present in the body. It measures allergic responses of the IgE antibodies to various items you might be allergic to, such as food allergies. Remember that ideally you aren't supposed to have food allergies because your body is supposed to digest food down to its smallest particles, which aren't allergenic.

Patch tests can be done to show the presence of delayed allergic reactions— those that usually cause skin rashes. The test is done by taping a bit of the possibly allergenic substance to the skin for about 48 hours. The dermatologist who does this kind of testing measures the amount of reaction on the skin.

Both respiratory and food allergens can be tested for the presence of an allergy.

- **Food Allergy Testing or Sensitivity Testing.** You can actually do your own allergy testing without having to see the doctor. There is a company called YORKTEST that provides you with information as to the top 36 most common food allergies and inhalation allergies. You need a blood sample taken, however, in order to do this test. You can also test for food allergies by doing what's called an elimination diet. You get rid of suspected food allergens in your diet for several months and see if your symptoms improve. You should have a doctor monitor you throughout the testing period. Finally, you can do blood tests that evaluate you for up to 113 food allergies. A pin prick amount of blood is tested against the allergen on a small card. If there is a food allergy, the reaction between the blood and the food allergen will be positive.

- **Live Blood Cell Analysis.** This is a test that involves putting a small amount of blood on a slide and covering the sample with a cover slip. The image is viewed under high power so that the doctor examining the slide can see changes in the red blood cells and white blood cells suggestive of the presence of pathogens, immune dysfunction, oxygen free radicals, pancreatic disorders, digestive disorders, liver problems, and oxidative stress on the body. The pathogens can be viruses, bacteria, parasites or fungi that have made their way into the bloodstream. Vitamin deficiencies, malnutrition, bodily stress, and mineral deficiencies can show changes in the blood that do not directly tell what's wrong but can be a good way of screening for the presence of diseases that can show up in the blood.

- **Amino Acid Analysis.** Remember that amino acids are the building blocks of protein and should be absorbed by the GI tract as individual amino acids. When made into proteins, they repair tissue, make antibodies, produce hormones (insulin, growth hormone, glucagon, etc.), produce enzymes that work inside the body and carry oxygen inside the red blood cells. Remember, too, that there are 8 essential amino acids and 12 that can be made using other molecules in the body. If you don't eat enough protein in your diet, you can become deficient in essential amino acids and the proteins they make. The test involves checking the amino acid content of a 24 hour urine collection and can check for the presence of leaky gut syndrome, heart disease, autism, anxiety diseases, behavioral conditions, chronic fatigue syndrome, fibromyalgia and various other digestive diseases.

These are the places you might consider going to in order to be evaluated for leaky gut syndrome. In the vast majority of cases, you can just send samples of urine, blood or stool to get your body tested for the disease.

Biolab. This is considered one of the best medical laboratories specializing in mineral analysis, environmental medicine, nutritional medicine, toxin analysis, fatty acid testing, pesticide analysis and environmental agent testing. They have learned to specialize in the various effects of a modern lifestyle on one's overall health. They have two tests which evaluate a person for leaky gut syndrome.

The first test is called a gut permeability profile. It utilizes a specific substance known as polyethylene glycol which is taken in by mouth. It is not absorbed by the gut in normal humans. A 6 hour urine is taken and evaluated for the presence of polyethylene glycol or PEG 400. If there is a great deal of polyethylene glycol in the urine, the gut must be leaky.

The other test is a test which measures the amount of short-chain polypeptides about 1-2 hours after eating a meal that is high in protein. If the protein is incompletely digested due to leaky gut syndrome, there will be a number of short chain polypeptides in the blood that ideally shouldn't be there. These short chain polypeptides will mimic the activity of cytokines and normal hormones, disrupting the biochemical milieu.

Remember you need a doctor's prescription to be able to do the testing.

The Diagnostic Clinic by Dr. Rajendra Sharma. This clinic does the polyethylene glycol test in much the same way as the Biolab. The clinic requests that you empty your urine before doing the test and then asks you to drink the polyethylene glycol. It is expected that a very small number of the polyethylene glycol molecules will enter the bloodstream under normal circumstances and when a large amount of molecules are found in the urine, it is indicative of leaky gut syndrome. The laboratory will send you a package containing the polyethylene glycol solution and a collection device for the urine, which is to be lastly collected 6 hours after ingestion of the substance. The test is available, once it has arrived at the facility, within 7 days of reception.

Another test for leaky gut syndrome is called the gut fermentation study and looks for the presence of Candida (yeast) within the gut. The patient must drink a sugary drink or take a capsule containing a sugary substance and then the blood is evaluated for the presence of alcohols, which are present because of the fermentation of the absorbed sugars by yeast. This is also a test that is useful for testing the body for the presence of dietary fiber, the presence of hypoglycemia and the presence of dysbiosis (having bad bacteria within the gut flora).

The lab can also do food allergy testing using the food allergy cellular test. It tests for inflammatory compounds that are emitted from the body's white blood cells because there is an offending allergenic food. Remember that food allergies can both cause leaky gut syndrome and can be an effect of it.

Another test is called the Bioresonance Food Intolerance Test. It checks for food intolerances using a special computer called a "bioresonance computer". A special nutritionist is used to interpret the data on food allergies.

The lab can also do a BioHit test, which is a measure of stomach acid production. If there is a lack of good digestion, molecules of food will be partially digested and will trigger food allergies. The BioHit test measures the amount of acid in the stomach through a blood test. Low acid production can mean leaky gut syndrome.

An ELISA/ACT test can be done to check for hidden food allergies and chemical hypersensitivities. It will be positive for these conditions if you have leaky gut syndrome. It can pick up mercury toxicity from mercury-containing dental amalgams, which can then be treated by removing the amalgams.

If you suspect that you have leaky gut syndrome or have one of the diseases noted at the top of this chapter, the cause could be leaky gut and you will want to go further by having one of these tests available to you in order to evaluate your condition. As noted, not all labs will run these types of tests; however, a lab that specializes in environmental medicine or toxic substances will usually have a division that does testing for gut permeability.

Chapter 5: Keeping the Gastrointestinal System in Balance

Restoring gut balance to rid the body of leaky gut syndrome means to get rid of gut dysbiosis or the presence of unhealthy bacteria in the gut milieu. Gut dysbiosis is one of the things that can perpetuate the cycle of leaky gut syndrome.

Bowel Dysbiosis

Dysbiosis of the gut happens when you take antibiotics for an illness and the antibiotic wipes out the normal bacteria that live in the small and especially the large intestine. These healthy bacteria aid in digestion and do not cause inflammation of the intestinal mucosa as do the "bad" bacteria.

While there are times that you must take an antibiotic for something, you need to consider that it could disrupt your intestinal bacterial milieu. The intestinal bacteria and yeast become unbalanced, leading to fermentation occurring in the gut. There can be an increase in the amount of mucus produced by the gut in response to the dangerous bacteria in an attempt to flush them out. There are unabsorbed and only partially digested carbohydrates in the mucus as well as toxic byproducts of mucus formation, leading to "mucus colitis", which manifests itself as chronic diarrhea.

Besides antibiotic use, which destroys healthy bacteria, you can get bowel or gut dysbiosis by having a parasitic infection, such as an overgrowth of Candida albicans. If your digestion is not optimal or your diet is poor, you can have an increase in the unhealthy bacteria in your gut.

Restoring the Gut Milieu through Diet

The diet that best works for gut dysbiosis involves some things you may not have thought of. One of these is raw vegetable juice.

This means that you use chemically free raw and organically-grown veggies and run them through a juicer. You should aim to drink about a pint per day.

Carrot juice is considered the best along with celery juice, which is low in its glycemic index. Barley grass juice will alkalinize the body and will be very beneficial. Raw beet root juice is good for the blood and helps the cells oxygenate better. You can also add a mixture of carrots, beet root, celery, broccoli, parsley and radish to make a health juice that is good for the bowel dysbiosis problem.

Raw eggs are an excellent protein source but must come from chickens that are organically grown, free range and free from Salmonella. Make sure you keep them in the cupboard and not in the refrigerator. They will keep in a cupboard at 20 degrees Celsius for about 2 weeks. They can be eaten one at a time or they can be mixed with vegetable juice. You should eat about 3-4 eggs per day to get the right amount of protein in your diet. They are an easy to digest protein and can be eaten by adults, the elderly, and children alike. Fresh raw eggs are excellent for the immune system. They provide raw fats and is one of the most protein-containing foods known.

Avocados have an extremely low glycemic index and contain helpful fats. They are almost considered a complete food and would be complete when combined with barley grass juice. Another healthy food is called "cold-pressed" honey. This is honey that has not been heated above 40 degrees Celsius. The healthy enzymes in honey are good for you and it satisfies your sweet tooth when added to avocadoes. Avocadoes can be eaten plain or blended with other vegetable juices, with honey to taste.

Raw milk is excellent for the bloodstream and blood products. It helps to make new blood cells and is considered a complete food. You need to find milk that is unpasteurized and raw, perhaps from a dairy farm. Pasteurized milk that has come from cows that have been raised with hormones is probably not the best milk to drink when compared to raw milk from healthy, unpasteurized, free grazing cows. If you have trouble with cow's milk, then go on to goat's milk that is raw and unpasteurized or sheep's milk. Sheep's milk can usually only be obtained directly from a farm that raises sheep. Raw milk of any kind can only usually be found at certain licensed farms. If it is quick-frozen, it can retain many of its healthy enzymes.

A healthy diet to turn around leaky gut syndrome is that which allows you to consume raw meat. Tenderize the meat in lime juice for a few hours and serve it at 37 degrees Celsius but not above 40 degrees Celsius. Soak it in sea water or add Celtic Sea Salt for flavor but do not add regular salt. You can purchase clean sea water through companies that sell a sun concentrate of sea water. Raw fish can be tenderized in lime juice or lemon juice and eat it raw. Tuna and salmon are best eaten raw, especially sliced and seasoned with olive oil and sea salt. Warmed rainbow trout that is still raw but warmed gently is extremely palatable and is healthy to eat.

Salads are also healthy to eat but you need to put in the salad highly valuable vegetables like water cress, tomatoes and spinach leaves. They contain healthy vegetables that are good for your gut. Water is also considered extremely valuable for the treatment of dysbiosis. You need to have de-chlorinated water that is considered well-filtered spring water or mineral water. You should use osmotically-filtered water or distilled water. You can add small amount of minerals to the water as well as a small amount of medicinal seawater concentrate and molasses.

Supplements that help treat Gut Dysbiosis

There are several supplements that help get rid of gut dysbiosis. They include the following:

- **Organic Silicon**. It helps detoxify the immune system and aids cellular regeneration in cases where the cells have been damaged. It is also used to treat psoriasis and certain types of arthritis. Anywhere there is pain and inflammation, organic silicon seems to work.

- **Zell Immunocomplex**. This product contains "Zell oxygen" as well as several nutrients, including antioxidants, trace minerals, and beta glucans.

- **Probiotics**. We will talk more about probiotics later in the next section. Suffice it to say that a good probiotic can reestablish a healthy biotic state in the GI tract.

Probiotics

Bacteria are plentiful in your body and, in fact, you have twenty times more bacteria in your body than there are cells in your body. There are billions of bacterial cells within your body and most reside within your gut. They are important to your health and wellbeing because they help digest food you cannot digest yourself.

Probiotics are healthy and "friendly" bacteria in your gut because they keep you from having an overgrowth of unhealthy bacteria and yeast within your system. They help you, in a sense, fight off diseases. Under normal circumstances, about 85 percent of the bacteria in your large bowel are considered "friendly" bacteria. They prevent bad bugs like E. coli and Salmonella from taking over and causing disease in the gut. The remaining 15 percent of bacteria are unfriendly but our bodies can handle them because they are kept in check by the good bacteria.

Probiotic as a word actually means "for life". This is because these organisms are helpful to the preservation of life. Scientifically, a probiotic means that the substance is a live microbial supplement that beneficially affects the host organism by improving the intestinal milieu. Probiotics are helpful for the immune system because they favorably change the gut micro-ecology so that the unfriendly bacteria can't gain a strong presence within the body. When probiotics are not around, the bad bacteria set up an inflammatory response within the body. Probiotics also lessen the risk of high cholesterol by lowering the body's cholesterol level.

Probiotics taken as supplements are excellent for yeast overgrowth. Candida yeast species can set up an overgrowth of yeast/fungi that cause leaky gut syndrome. Probiotics also help treat other bodily infections such as vaginal yeast infections and athlete's foot. There are more than 400 species of healthy, symbiotic bacteria that normally should inhabit the intestinal tract. There are things in your diet and other things you can do to disrupt this normal milieu.

The two things that create intestinal dysbiosis or disruption of the intestinal bacteria the most are chlorine and sodium fluoride. Both of these chemicals are found in ordinary pre-treated city water. So, if you drink water from the tap or at restaurants, you are likely getting water that is damaging to your gut flora.

Other things to consider as adversely affecting the gut flora are antibiotics, certain other drugs, and oral contraceptives. Some can adversely affect the intestinal flora and others can directly damage the intestinal wall. When there are too many bad bacteria and not enough good bacteria, you get excessive amounts of gas, constipation, bloating, toxicity from the intestinal contents, and poor absorption of healthy nutrients.

Taking Probiotics

You need to take a probiotic supplement that is enteric coated so the stomach doesn't destroy the bacteria or take supplements that contain protective spores that do not blossom into bacteria until they pass through the stomach and into the intestine, when the environment is right.

Probiotics are helpful in inhibiting the excess growth of harmful bacteria that can cause digestive distress. They can also improve the absorption of vitamins and the digestion of the food we take in. They help stimulate the body's normal defensive immune system and help in the formation of vitamins the body actually needs.

What, besides supplements, are other ways we can get probiotics into our system? We can eat live yogurt cultures, Japanese Miso, some types of cheeses and Tempeh. These have some moderate probiotic activity within the gut. Unfortunately, it is not always clear how much probiotic bacteria you're getting in the above foods and how many of the bacteria will survive the harsh, acidic environment of the stomach to reach the colon. In addition, foods like garlic, onions and bananas have probiotic activity but again, the action is mild and unpredictable.

When choosing a probiotic, make sure it is enteric coated so it will survive the environment of the stomach and will open up and release healthy bacteria in the small intestines and colon. The stomach area is completely sterile due to its extremely acidic environment. Under ideal situations of normal stomach activity, both the good and bad bacteria survive. If an enteric coated product containing probiotic bacteria survive, then they can populate the small and large intestine.

Common probiotic bacteria are Lactobacillus and other lactic acid bacteria, Bifidobacteria and Acidophilus as well as some healthy yeast. These are contained in pill form, enteric caplet form, capsules and within foods like yogurts.

Rotation Diets

Rotation diets are good for people who have food allergies. It involves a way of eating certain biologically related foods all on the same day and then holding off from those foods for a minimum of 4 days before trying to eat them again. Rotation diets are able to prevent allergic reactions to new foods.

Foods eaten in a repetitive fashion can trigger food allergies because you are always exposed to them, especially if you are afflicted with leaky gut syndrome. It also allows you to eat foods to which you are allergic. If you simply remove the foods to which you are allergic, you will eventually develop an allergy to the foods used to replace the one's you were allergic to in the first place.

A rotation diet lets you eat certain foods to which there is a mild or borderline allergic potential that would make you sick if you at them every day or oftener than every 4 days. Remember, too, that your level of stress will negatively impact your food allergies so you must be sure to rest as much as you need to and modify your diet toward less allergenic foods when you are sick or have an infection.

Rotation diets take practice, and careful attention to what you are eating. Like any kind of dietary change, you need to make sure you pay attention in the beginning, knowing that it will gradually become second nature after a while. There are several kinds of "free" foods that can be eaten on any given day. There are also some spices that are considered "free" so that you can make sure your food is edible. Take a look at the Ultimate Food Allergy Cookbook and other cookbooks that offer advice on the rotation diet so that those of you with leaky gut syndrome can enjoy foods in specific ways without experiencing allergic symptoms, regardless of what those symptoms might be.

The extra foods you eat do not have a specific day attached to them, such as "chicken and rice" day but still must be written down when eaten so that you don't eat them for another four days or more. Foods that have mild allergic potential can be eaten more often than foods that have a highly allergic potential.

The diet needs to be modified according to your symptoms. If you find that certain foods are causing an allergic reaction more than you expected, put them in the "elimination" column for a while and put in their place more familiar food families or the extra foods. On the days off a food, your antibody levels gradually drop so that you can eventually eat the food again.

You don't need to suffer on this type of diet. Instead, you can freeze special desserts and foods that freeze well so you can take them out for special occasions. Make sure you make the foods yourself so you know it contains nothing allergenic. You need as much variety as you possibly can so your mental health is restored by the eating process. You will be repeating foods every four to five days but you can change the foods around so that they aren't in the same form each and every day.

Travelling may be difficult while on a rotation diet. During such times, it is probably better to stay with foods to which you know you are not allergic. As processed sugar is bad for those with leaky gut syndrome, you should avoid foods high in sugar. You shouldn't have to get picky about how much you eat because if you're eating well, your weight will stabilize, even with the allergies you have.

Chapter 6: Treating LGS with Nutritional Supplements

Because allopathic medical science does not often recognize leaky gut syndrome, there aren't many allopathic treatments to treat this type of condition. Fortunately, there are several nutritional supplements that treat this disease. Let's take a look at some of them:

- **Probiotics** can correct the problem of leaky gut syndrome by replacing bad bacteria with beneficial bacteria. The probiotics can be taken in by certain foods but it is best taken as an enteric coated supplement that provides the gut with healthy bacteria that do not produce the toxins that unhealthy bacteria produce.

- **Following a Leaky Gut diet and taking healthy supplements** can help digestion and can reverse leaky gut syndrome. A leaky gut diet is low in allergenic foods, high in nutrients and does not irritate the lining of the gut. Avoid refined sugars, which are currently consumed at a rate of 150 pounds per person per year. Refined sugar contributes to obesity, offers no nutritional benefit and lowers immunity. It also irritates the lining of the intestinal mucosa. The heart, liver and pancreas are overloaded when you take in too much sugar. Remember that sugars are contained in high fructose corn syrup, sucrose, glucose, and glucose-sucrose.

Cut out regular soda pop and diet soda pop. Each can of regular soda pop contains about 10 teaspoons of sugar per can. There is artificial dye, artificial flavorings, and caffeine in these liquids. The carbonation of these beverages can lead to bone mineral loss and osteoporosis.

Avoid enriched white flours. The fiber has been removed from these food products and they are highly refined with synthetic vitamin B's added back to the flour. It otherwise offers no significant healthy benefit and can contribute to leaky gut syndrome.

Avoid alcohol and caffeinated beverages. Alcohol is an irritant to the intestinal lining when you drink too much and caffeine also irritates the intestinal mucosa. Caffeine dehydrates the body. You should drink much more plain water than these beverages.

Certain drugs damage the intestinal mucosa. They lead to leaky gut syndrome. The worst drugs to take include NSAIDS like naproxen, aspirin, and ibuprofen, and steroidal drugs like hydrocortisone and prednisone will contain irritants that bother the intestinal wall. Other drugs to be careful of include antibiotics, chemotherapeutic agents, nicotine and antacids.

• **Improving your digestion** will help leaky gut syndrome. You need to start by eating smaller bites of food and by chewing food well so that your oral digestive enzymes can begin to break down food adequately. Take a digestive enzyme that will improve your digestion further. This can be problematic if you take digestive enzymes containing protease and also have a pancreas problem or those that contain HCl or hydrochloric acid and already have stomach ulcers.

Put as much soluble fiber and insoluble fiber in your diet. Insoluble fiber provides bulk to your stools and soluble fiber gets rid of toxic wastes and excess cholesterol from your diet. Add probiotics to this healthy balance of fiber and you will have a reduced risk of leaky gut syndrome.

Quit drinking large amounts of cold fluid with your dinner as it dilutes out the stomach acid and destroys the activity of vitamins. If you drink small amounts of water that has freshly squeezed lemon juice in the water (drink less than a half cup), you can have better digestion, especially if you eat a lot of protein in your diet or make too little stomach acid. Don't overeat because this makes digestion last too long, makes for incomplete digestion, stresses out the liver and can lead to negative bacteria within the colon.

- **Nutrients to eat for leaky gut syndrome** include those containing L-glutamine, found in the intestinal tract and that promotes healing of the GI tract. Try products that contain slippery elm, citrus bioflavanoids, and marshmallow root. They heal the intestinal lining and help with the reduction of inflammation. Also try the healing powers of aloe vera juice. Omega 3 essential fatty acids, commonly seen in cold water fish, help heal the intestinal lining and improve the function of the immune system. Multivitamins with minerals help those with leaky gut syndrome get the nutrients many are missing in their poor diets.

Supplements that contain vitamin A are healthy because they contain the backbone for the production of IgA, which are the protective surface antibodies of the GI tract. Vitamin A also maintains a healthy GI tract, soothing inflammation and leading to a healthy mucosa. It is best taken as an emulsion because it coats the lining of the intestines better. You can take up to 25,000 IU per day of Vitamin A and still have it be a healthy amount.

The Zinc in your diet is helpful for the growth and healing of damaged cells. Zinc is vital to the health of the intestinal lining because these are cells that are rapidly turned over. The leaky gut syndrome seen in Crohn's disease patients is healed through the consumption of zinc. Zinc is a common deficiency in leaky gut syndrome. If you are deficient in zinc, you need to consume about 50-80 mg per day. Don't take in excess of 100 mf per day as this amount can inhibit the immune system. Take about one milligram of copper for each 15 milligrams of zinc so you won't get copper deficiency from taking in all that zinc.

N-Acetyl Glucosamine is an amino sugar that contains a combination of sugar and an amino acid. It helps secrete the mucus that protects the gastrointestinal lining from dangerous pathogens and toxins.

N-Acetyl Cysteine (NAC) is related to the amino acid called cysteine and is a potent antioxidant and detoxifying agent. It helps make the body's glutathione, which is great for detoxifying toxins. N-Acetyl Cysteine gets rid of toxins produced by the overgrowth of bad bacteria and intestinal yeast. If you take a probiotic along with NAC, it can help establish the healthy bacteria in the gut. It helps the liver in its detoxifying power and provides sulfur molecules that go on to make powerful enzymes in the liver. By helping the liver function better, it gives the GI tract a rest so that it can heal. The dose is 500 to 1000 mg taken twice daily.

Seacure is a product made by Proper Nutrition, Inc., that is made by white fish pellets that are partially digested by micro-organisms from the sea. The product contains small polypeptides that help leaky gut syndrome. The polypeptides help heal the intestinal wall by acting as growth factors. It is known to help people with leaky gut syndrome, irritable bowel syndrome, ulcerative colitis and Crohn's disease.

- **Environmental things to avoid** if you have leaky gut syndrome include:

  o Certain drugs like NSAIDS, pain relievers, and antacids
  o Alcohol
  o Caffeine
  o Environmental toxins like pesticides or residue of pesticides on certain foods
  o Food additives, including food colors, food preservatives and artificial flavorings
  o Spicy foods, which irritate the lining of the stomach and intestines
  o Yeast that makes toxic alcohols in the GI tract that damage the intestinal lining

- **Reducing stress** is another way to decrease the over-activeness of the GI tract as seen with leaky gut syndrome. The brain contains neurohormones that act on both the brain and the GI tract. Stress affects these neurochemicals and, in fact, the brain and the GI tract are so closely connected that when you feel stressed out, it is common to have gastrointestinal symptoms. Your brain affects the amount of blood flow to the digestive tissues and, without them, they are deprived of oxygen, blood sugar, and essential nutrients. Chronic stress means that you don't make enough digestive mucus and you are more likely to get irritable bowel syndrome and leaky gut syndrome.

It's a good idea to practice relaxation techniques when trying to recover from leaky gut syndrome. Some very effective techniques for reducing stress include self-hypnosis, meditation, prayer, biofeedback, breathing techniques, and listening to soothing music.

- **Taking in fructooligosaccharides (FOS)** in your diet seems to help leaky gut syndrome. These are short chain polysaccharides in which the major sugar is fructose instead of glucose. They add fiber to the diet and are not digested because we lack the necessary enzymes to digest them. Healthy bacteria such as Bifidobacteria contain the enzymes to break down FOS and this promotes growth of these healthy bacteria. It has the natural sweetness of sugar but no calories. You can find FOS in artichokes, asparagus, onions, leeks, bananas, burdock, soybeans and chicory. FOS is also manufactured to be put along with probiotics in order to promote their growth and development in the gut.

- **Vitamin E** is a healthy antioxidant that protects gut tissue from being acted on by oxygen free radicals. These oxygen free radicals can endanger cells that line the GI tract and can become a self-perpetuating cycle. Antioxidants can also help reverse the aging process. You need Vitamin E in order to keep your immune system very strong and to help it act against the bacteria and viruses that are so dangerous in leaky gut syndrome.

The best way to get vitamin E is to eat it in healthy foods. Some healthy foods that contain vitamin E include nuts, vegetable oils, sunflower seeds, spinach, broccoli and fortified breakfast cereals, fortified juices, margarine that is fortified to contain vitamin E and sandwich spreads. High doses of vitamin E are dangerous so you need to avoid taking high dose supplements of the vitamin.

- **Pycogenol** is a natural plant extract that comes from the bark of a pine tree growing along the coastline of southwestern France. It contains procyanidins and bioflavonoids that together have several important properties in the treatment of leaky gut syndrome. It contains anti-inflammatory properties and is a strong antioxidant, allowing healing of the gut tissue by dilating blood vessels near the gut wall. The dilated blood vessels allow for more nutrients to aid in gut healing. It also binds selectively to elastin and collagen.

- **Vitamin B12** is another vitamin important for digestion. It often comes as a part of the vitamin B complex of vitamins. It is vital for methylation of proteins and for DNA synthesis. It is released by stomach acid when protein is introduced into the stomach. Then B12 connects to intrinsic factor and is absorbed into the blood in the small intestines. Vitamin B12 is stored nicely in the liver but, if intrinsic factor is missing, there can eventually be anemia called pernicious anemia.

Typical nutritional supplements for leaky gut syndrome can be taken in the following doses:

- Vitamin B5—5 mg per day

- Vitamin B6—50 mg per day

- B Complex Vitamins—50 mg twice daily

- Vitamin C—1000 to 3000 mg per day, taking lower doses if there is stomach or bowel discomfort

- Vitamin E—take 2000 international units per day

- PABA—take up to 2000 to 3000 mg per day for six months or so

- Lactobacillus acidophilus—take one to two capsules or one teaspoon daily

- DHEA—take 0.5-10 mg per day, depending on your herbalist's recommendation

- L-Glutathione—take 75 milligrams twice daily

- Coenzyme Q—take 320 milligrams daily

- Pycogenol—take 50 milligrams three times per day

- N acetyl cysteine—250 mg per day

- Selenium—100 mg per day.

There are many herbal and natural remedies for the treatment of leaky gut syndrome and more can be expected as research discovers more and more about the condition and the actions of herbal remedies. Those nutritional supplements or herbal remedies that increase mucus production in the gut, are anti-inflammatory and naturally anti-bacterial and anti-viral seem to have the best effectiveness

against leaky gut syndrome and are considered the most promising remedies to try.

Always talk to a good herbalist if you are
considering using an herbal remedy for leaky
gut syndrome as they have good information
as to how much to take and which is the best
form to take it in.

Putting it All Together: What you should do for Leaky Gut Syndrome

There are general guidelines you should be
following for the management of your life
with leaky gut syndrome. These guidelines
offer you a way to run your life that keeps you
in charge of the disease.

- **Reduce the number of medicines you are taking.** If your doctor allows it, you should get rid of any medications that might be contributing to your getting leaky gut syndrome. Your doctor is the best person to give you this advice. You might be able to come up with some herbal remedies that do the same thing without the harsh side effects on your system.

- **Use only natural and organic bath products, cosmetics and cleaning products.** Look for product that contain Sodium lauryl sulfate and avoid using products containing it. This product was originally an industrial grease remover and floor cleansing agent. As our bodies take up nearly 60 percent of all lotions, creams and liquids rubbed into it every day, you need to make sure that you don't give it anything dangerous or allergenic.

Sodium lauryl sulfate strips the skin of the protective oils it secretes to keep itself healthy and waterproof. This allows the skin to dry out and allows certain products that are unhealthy to get into the skin. Sodium lauryl sulfate has been found in studies to be linked to getting cataracts and to allow nitrates into the body, which are cancer-causing agents. Other products for cleansing the body contain parabens, drying alcohol and other chemicals that can lead to an allergic reaction.

- **Eat small yet frequent meals.** This can allow the gut to better handle the load given to it so that you don't give the gut a large load to handle. Eating too much at one time leads to poor digestion and poor absorption.

- **Only eat when you are hungry.** If you eat only when hungry and eat until full, you can provide your body with what it needs without overloading the gut.

- **Handle stress the best way you can.** Take up meditation, Qi Gong, yoga or Reiki. These are ways you can tackle the stress in your life by practicing time-held traditional methods of relaxation, which can, in turn, help improve your symptoms of leaky gut syndrome.

- **Practice Dry Skin Brushing.** This is a technique that is used to cleanse the lymph system. You do it before a bath or shower, brushing always toward the center portion of your body. Sweep the entire body before bathing.

- **Practice coffee enemas.** These are well known to clean out the liver and helps detoxify the body. You need to do coffee enemas several times per day until the toxins of the body are gone and you feel better. It may take several days of coffee enemas to improve your system. It gives the liver a rest so it isn't so overwhelmed. Have a healthcare provider show you how to do it before attempting the procedure on yourself.

- **Sleep, Sleep and Sleep.** As adults, you need around 8-9 hours of sleep per night. Too many people don't get enough sleep and this can weaken the immune system, drop your temperature, lower your white blood cell count and decrease growth hormone production. Make sure you go to bed by 11 pm, even if you don't feel tired.

- **Try Acidophilus Pearls™.** These are pearls of helpful probiotics that aid digestion and coat the intestines with healthy bacteria. There is a natural coating on the pearls that allow the acidophilus to make it past the harsh environment of the stomach.

Chapter 7: Treating & Preventing LGS with Stress Management

It is well known that stress can bring on leaky gut syndrome and can make leaky gut syndrome worse. It stands to reason then, that those who practice stress relief can improve their symptoms of leaky gut syndrome and can prevent it from happening in the first place.

As mentioned in earlier chapters, the GI tract is perhaps the most responsive body system when it comes to brain and stress influences. The gut contains neurohormone receptors, which are receptors that respond to hormones released by the brain. Some researchers call the gut the "second brain" because brain chemicals seem to be very active in the GI tract.

What this means is that stress in the brain strongly affects stress in the gut. When you're under stress, the blood is washed away from the digestive system toward the skeletal muscle in what scientists know is the "fight or flight" response. This deprives the GI tract of glucose, oxygen and essential chemical nutrients. If you're chronically stressed out, your digestive system is chronically starved and adequate amounts of mucus cannot be made. This leads to leaky gut syndrome and, in some cases, irritable bowel syndrome.

Some doctors feel as though stress is the number one thing that leads to leaky gut syndrome and that stress reduction is the number one way to manage the disease. The trick is to learn how to put the brain into the alpha state (with a brain wave frequency of 8-12 Hertz) or into the theta state, with a brain wave frequency of 4-8 Hertz. Instead it is delta waves that are associated with stress. This has a brain wave frequency of 2-4 Hertz.

Stress relief may be as simple as getting enough sleep, resting when necessary, eating healthy foods at the right time of day and having a low stress job. You may actively need to learn about relaxation and take on practices that can help you live a stress-free life or at least to handle stressors in your life with ease.

There are several different kinds of stress-relieving activities you can partake in that will actively help you improve your stress levels. Exactly which activity you pick depends on your physical activity level, flexibility and personal interest. Let's look at some excellent ways to reduce stress, change your neurohormone levels and improve the circulation and health of your gut.

Self-Hypnosis

This can be done by people that have no ability to be physically active. It uses traditional methods of hypnosis but applies these techniques to you for medical and therapeutic reasons. You can best learn self-hypnosis by being hypnotized by an expert and by learning ways to repeat the hypnotic trance yourself. Everyone has different ways to put themselves into a hypnotic state. One typical way is to close your eyes, think pleasant thoughts and count backwards from 10 to 1.

Self-hypnosis can help you get rid of stress, nervousness, anxiety and depression. It requires regular practice at least one to two times daily. Once hypnotized, tell yourself you are calm, at peace, well-rested and well. Breathe deeply, in through your nose and out through your mouth. This increases the amount of blood flow you get to your brain, inducing relaxation of the gut wall, relaxation of muscles and a peaceful sense of wellbeing. You give yourself positive suggestions that can heal damaged tissue, give you stress relief and substitute negative self-thoughts with positive self-thoughts.

The biggest benefit of self-hypnosis is that you can do this on your own without having to see a therapist or hypnotist every week or even every day. Self-hypnosis can be a powerful way to improve your life and rid yourself of leaky gut syndrome. As long as you learn the technique from a trained professional, you should be able to continue on in your own fashion.

Biofeedback

Biofeedback involves a technique where your mind actively works to change bodily functions, such as your heart rate, etc., with thinking. It requires in the beginning that you be hooked up to sensors that can help you concentrate and focus on things such as heart rate, skin moisture and other bodily sensations. You learn to relax and slow your body down so that you can put yourself into a state of complete relaxation. It gives you the chance to use your mind in order to control your body. You use feedback from your body signals in order to put your mind in a state that perfects the healing process.

Biofeedback can be used for many things including, asthma, stress, anxiety, chemotherapy effects, GI symptoms, heart problems, hypertension, incontinence, irritable colon, physical pain, and Raynaud's disease. In athletes, it is used to boost physical performance.

People seem to respond so well to biofeedback because it isn't invasive, it can reduce the need for many medications, it is a good treatment for those who can't take medications because of their leaky gut, and it helps people take charge of their physical health and well-being.

Biofeedback usually is something that should be taught by a licensed and certified biofeedback training specialist. Some biofeedback specialists are good for some diseases, while other biofeedback specialists are good for other diseases. Make sure you ask the biofeedback technician if they are certified or licensed and what training they have. Ask them how many sessions you'll need before you can go it alone without the actual sensors helping you.

In biofeedback sessions in the beginning, you will have sensors placed that monitor your skin temperature, your level of muscle tension, your brain waves or your heart rate. A beeping sound or light flashing will signal when you're not in the right range and further relaxation and deep thought will bring you back into the right range. In the beginning, the sessions last about 30-60 minutes in length. It may take up to 50 sessions in severe cases but even 10 sessions can make all the difference in the world when it comes to leaky gut syndrome or irritable bowel symptoms.

There are several types of biofeedback techniques, all of which have some potential to reverse leaky gut syndrome. These include those that measure:

- **Your muscle tension**. It uses an EMG to provide information about how tense your muscles are.

- **Your skin temperature**. This uses thermal feedback sensors that provide you with ways to bring up your body temperature. The temperature normally lowers with stress so you can use the body temperature sensors to relieve stress.

- **Your sweat gland activity**. These include the use of galvanic skin responses to alert you when you're excessively sweating, which indicates stress and anxiety.

- **Your heartbeat**. This uses commercially available EKG leads to detect your heart rate. When you can control your heart rate, you control your blood pressure and your stress levels goes way down. Eventually, you can control your heart rate on your own.

Feedback therapy can involve you being attached to big computers or small hand-held devices that give you constant feedback on your heart rate or other body stimuli. You eventually learn what it takes to do this on your own so you don't need the feedback anymore. You can reduce stress at any point you feel like you need some stress relief. It can improve your leaky gut syndrome after less than a month of therapy.

Meditation

Meditation is an excellent thing to try if you suffer from anxiety, tension, worry or stress. It is the preferred technique for stress relief by millions of people worldwide. Its popularity is made more so by the fact that it is easy to do, inexpensive and requires no special equipment. Meditation can be practiced anywhere, from on the bus, at work, in your own bed or while taking a walk. Meditation has been practiced by different cultures for thousands of years and was once said to be a way to connect with all that was sacred or mystical. In today's time, it has excellent uses in the reduction of stress and the promotion of relaxation.

When meditating, you can achieve a much deeper state of relaxation than you can in real life. Your attention is focused and you can easily throw away thoughts that normally jumble your mind. It's these jumbled thoughts that cause the stress. Take away stress and you have better health and an increase in emotional wellbeing.

The beneficial effects of meditation include gaining a sense of peacefulness and calm, finding balance in your life, and in improving stress-related diseases such as leaky gut syndrome. Meditation has a lasting effect on your body, improving your physical state up until you need to meditate again.

As you can see, meditation offers both emotional and physical benefits. Some of the emotional benefits include:

- Improvement in self-awareness

- Having a better perspective on things that normally stress you out

- Building stress management skills

- Finding a focus on the present instead of on things you can't yet control or happened in the past

- Having a reduction in your negative emotions

Meditation has marvelous effects on physical illnesses, including leaky gut syndrome. By reducing your stress level, you also have no problems handling stressors that come your way. This changes the hormone levels of your body so you reduce the neurochemicals pathways that seem to be a part of leaky gut syndrome.

Other physical conditions believed to be helped by meditation include anxiety problems, allergies, cancer, asthma, binge eating, depression, tiredness, sleep disorders, substance abuse issues, chronic pain, high blood pressure, and heart disease. While meditation can't always take the place of conventional medical treatment, diseases like leaky gut syndrome that are related so strongly to stress can be greatly helped by meditation.

The goal of meditation is to achieve a relaxed mental and emotional state. There are fortunately many ways to do this and you can use any one of the several ways to relieve the symptoms of your leaky gut syndrome. Types of meditation include:

- **Mantra meditation**. This is a type of meditation in which you quietly or silently repeat a soothing or calming thought or word that removes distracting thoughts and allows you to relax into a deep and peaceful state. Stress flows away from the body and you feel better after a meditation session.

- **Guided meditation**. This is a type of meditation also called guided imagery. You use visualization by meditating on mental images of places you've been to or would like to go to that are particularly relaxing and soothing. Imagine how the place smells, looks, sounds and feels. You can use an audiotape at first in order to really visualize the calm and peaceful place. Then you imagine your body completely well within that place. It soothes and calms your mind and body.

- **Mindfulness meditation**. This involves being completely and totally aware of the present moment. You accept yourself and your circumstances for what they are and you intuit your experiences while staying in the moment. Practice deep breathing that is even and soothing. Observe the thoughts going through your head but don't judge them. Let your emotional being just be.

- **Transcendental Meditation**. This involves the use of a mantra, which is a word, phrase or sound that is repeated silently so that your consciousness becomes aware and you find yourself avoiding any thought so that you have a state that is perfectly still with the highest degree of consciousness.

There are stress-reducing techniques that involve relaxation through movement. Most of these have Asian origins and are great for people who are into movement and want to relieve stresses in their life at the same time. They are also great forms of exercise.

- **Qi gong**. This form of meditative exercise is pronounced "chee gung" and is a type of Chinese energy meditation. It uses gentle movements, breathing techniques and meditation all together in order to cleanse the body, strengthen the mind and body and allow the chi to circulate. It leads to stress-relief, relaxation, better health and improved vitality. People with leaky gut syndrome are more relaxed and feel much better than those who did not practice Qi Gong. It makes for a tranquil state of mind and involves doing inner work and guiding energy. This is a practice that has been popular in China as far back as 2500 years ago. In some ways, it is related to the Chinese practice of Tai chi.

- **Tai chi**. This is a form of Chinese martial arts that involves the use of very purposeful, yet gentle movements that gracefully guide the practitioner through a series of specific movement patterns. Breathing is deep and purposeful with stress relief gotten through the use of regular breathing and steady movements. Those who want some physical activity with their relaxation exercises would do much better with an activity like Tai Chi.

- **Yoga**. Yoga is an ancient form of exercise that involves putting the body into various relaxing postures while practicing breathing forms that relax the body and mind. It is a great stress-reliever and, by requiring balance and concentration, it clears the mind of other stressors that can get in the way of good health. Each session takes from 30-60 minutes and usually goes from mild relaxation exercises, through more energizing exercises and winds up with deep relaxation exercises/poses that ultimately reduce stress and make you feel more centered.

How does meditation work?

As you can see, meditation can take many forms and there are forms of meditation that will work better for you than others. Try doing one kind that involves simple relaxation and breathing techniques and experiment with another form that involves physical activity to see which one works best.

Meditation has several elements, regardless of the type you use that works to de-stress your mind and body. Remember that you can use an instructor who helps you learn to meditate or you can practice these forms of meditation on your own. Let's take a look at the elements of meditation that make it so successful.

- **Focused attention**. By focusing your attention away from stressful events and toward a singular thought or idea, you free yourself from distractions and are more able to use your mind to tell your body to heal and to remind yourself to relax, even after the meditation session is over with. Breathing is a good thing to focus on as is a specific object, mantra or an image of something that pleases you.

- **Relaxed breathing techniques**. Your breathing should remain even and deep, using your diaphragm muscles to fill your lungs with life-giving oxygen. Your breathing should be deep enough that slow breathing still gives you the oxygen you need. Let your shoulders, neck muscles and upper chest muscles relax so that your breathing can be efficient and should help you concentrate and focus.

- **Find a quiet setting**. When you're first learning to meditate, you need to be able to find a quiet place with which to practice the art of meditation. Don't allow yourself to be distracted by cell phones, televisions or radio noise. Your bedroom or lounge might be the place to start. After a while, you will be much more adept at meditation in settings that are a little more chaotic and you'll find yourself able to meditate in the middle of rush hour traffic, when the kids are screaming or when your work day is overwhelming.

- **Find a comfortable position**. You can do meditative techniques while lying down, sitting, walking or in different poses as in yoga. The more comfortable your body is in, the better relaxed you will be and the less stress you will notice.

Finding Ways to Incorporate Meditation into Daily Life

Just the thought of meditation freaks people out. They think of ancient Chinese philosophers and those that eat greens and do colon cleanses. Meditation can actually improve your life and can be done in ways that are private and personal. You don't have to have meditation instructors in order to practice the various forms of meditation on your own. Meditation can be a formal event or an informal practice you do in the privacy of your home or as part of your daily routine. You just need quality time alone for the practice of meditation.

Doing meditation on your own involves the following steps:

- Learn how to breathe deeply and let your mind focus solely on your breathing. Listen to your breathing and concentrate on your state of mind as you breathe. Inhale and exhale as you learned to do, even if you're on the bus or making dinner. Return your focus to your breathing whenever your mind wanders.

- Do a total body scan while you breathe. Focus on all your body sensation and note areas of pain, tension, relaxed body areas and those that feel cool or warm. Imagine breathing warmth and relaxation into those body parts that feel cool or tense. Let your body relax as much as is physically possible.

- Repeat a simple mantra that can be secular or religious. You can say a quick prayer popular in Judaism or Christianity or use the "om" mantra common to Hinduism and other Eastern religions.

- Use meditation while you walk. It uses calories and is a healthy way to enjoy a relaxing situation. Walk in a forest setting, down the street in the city or even at the mall. Just breathe, relax, and let the rhythm of your feet carry your mind away to other places and times when you felt more relaxed and at ease. Concentrate on the rise and fall of your legs and feet as you place them on the ground.

- Use prayer in every setting that makes sense for you to do it. You can pray with your own words or use already written prayers from your own faith. Twelve step programs offer great prayers and self-help books often include prayers or mantras you can use for relaxation.

- Read poems of reflection in order to get in the mood to meditate. This can be accompanied by listening to sacred music, soothing spoken words or doing anything else you find relaxing. Share your personal reflections in a journal or on your computer so that you can discuss them with a friend or spiritual leader.

- Pay attention to the love and gratitude you feel for others or for your life in general. Weave this kind of gratitude into the thoughts you have throughout the day. When you meditate, focus on a sacred object or person, allowing yourself to be grateful for the love you feel and for the presence of the object or person in your life.

Don't every judge your skills toward meditation as your skills will only get better over time. It takes practice to meditate well and practice makes perfect. Your mind might wander during meditation at first but you will become more focused over time. Just gently bring your mind back into what you're supposed to be thinking of while you meditate.

Experiment with your meditation so you can find which type works best for you and which ones you enjoy doing the most. You can't go wrong with meditation if your heart is in it and you let yourself practice. Soon, you will be de-stressed and will feel considerably better.

Chapter 8: Treating LGS with Herbal Remedies

As there are no allopathic (traditional) medical treatments for leaky gut syndrome, you need to think about taking herbal remedies for your condition. Herbs that tackle inflammation, improve the immune system, heal the gut lining, or provide mucus to the gut lining are all considered to be good herbs for leaky gut syndrome.

Remember that leaky gut syndrome ultimately affects the entire body, from the joints to the skin to the nervous system. When the protective lining of the gut is adversely affected, pathogens and food molecules from the outside have an easy in to the inside and many different complications can occur. This means that you might find yourself taking herbal remedies that do not directly affect the leaky gut but affect the parts of the body that are strongly altered by the presence of leaky gut syndrome.

When the gut is inflamed, many of the normal carrier proteins found in the GI tract that help certain nutrients pass from the inside of the intestines to the bloodstream, deficiencies of minerals can exist. Magnesium deficiency can lead to symptoms of fibromyalgia, even in the presence of high magnesium intake by the patient. When magnesium is low, you can get muscle spasms and muscle pain similar to fibromyalgia.

Zinc deficiencies are also possible and can lead to elevated blood cholesterol, which can lead to atherosclerosis of the arteries, heart disease and stroke. Calcium deficiency can lead to osteoporosis. Even trace mineral deficiencies can occur, such as a deficiency to silicon, manganese and boron—all of which can lead to various bone disorders if the deficiency is severe enough.

Any herb that has antioxidant therapeutic effects can make a difference in leaky gut syndrome. Good natural antioxidants include natural carotenoids (vitamin A), quercetin, catechins, citrus-based hesperidins, rutin, grape seed extracts, bilberry and cysteine, also called N-acetyl cysteine. Some people get better using the amino acid methionine and L glutathione. Vitamin C is a healthy antioxidant that works great with people who have damaged blood vessels from inflammation or who have diseases like asthma and other allergies.

Some anti-inflammatory agents include coenzyme Q10, B complex vitamins, folic acid and vitamin B12. Selenium works great for inflammation and helps certain enzymes work better. Many plant enzymes work well to treat leaky gut syndrome, including those found in chlorella plants, barley greens, Spirulina, and kamut. These things are also found in bee pollen and in royal jelly.

You need to be aware of the fact that low stomach levels of hydrochloric acid can contribute to leaky gut syndrome by poor digestion of proteins, allowing polypeptides to enter the GI tract. This can happen with the taking of antacids, the taking of histamine-2 blockers like Zantac® and Tagamet®, or the taking of proton pump inhibitors like Prilosec®.

When the stomach acid gets low, then there is a lowering of the absorption of vitamin B12 and you get pernicious anemia. In order to treat it, you need injections of vitamin

B12 along with oral folate treatment. Stomach acid can be lowered not only through anti-ulcer medication but can be a hereditary thing.

Other good supplements for stomach acid depletion include glutamic acid, which is an amino acid, hydrochloride, betaine hydrochloride, pepsin, which is a digestive enzyme your body lacks in low acid conditions, lemon juice, apple cider vinegar, pantothenic acid (vitamin B5), "stomach bitters", vitamin C, organic PABA, which is para-aminobenzoic acid, and pyridoxine, also called vitamin B6. By improving the stomach acid content, it aids digestion of proteins into amino acids or short chain peptides that are further broken down in the small intestine—entering the bloodstream in its normal amino acid form.

The natural hormone DHEA is a good treatment for people who have autoimmune conditions as a result of leaky gut syndrome. It is found in human brains and is the precursor molecule to testosterone. It is a good hormone to take if you have obesity, physical fatigue, a lack of libido, food allergies of many types, stress, low blood sugar and many autoimmune diseases.

As mentioned, the carrier proteins to minerals are depleted in leaky gut syndrome, resulting in a reduction of magnesium in the body system despite taking in a lot of magnesium. It simply passes through the gut unchanged and unabsorbed. This can lead to severe mineral deficiency in the bones, muscle spasms and pain in the muscles.

Zinc deficiency is also a result of a lack of carrier protein to bring it into the bloodstream. Without zinc, you can suffer from hair loss that can proceed to complete baldness or even alopecia areata—an immune disease affecting the hair production.

The loss of carrier protein production in leaky gut syndrome affects the absorption of boron, silicone, manganese, calcium and copper. As mentioned, copper deficiency can lead to high cholesterol levels, while the other trace and non-trace minerals are necessary for proper bone density.

When health amino acids aren't absorbed in the system, then proteins necessary for blood osmotic pressure aren't present and you can get edema, inflammation and tissue swelling as the fluid leaches out of the bloodstream that doesn't have the proper proteins to keep the fluid in the arteries and veins. Carrier proteins are necessary for the uptake of many vitamins and protein-based nutrients. Without the carrier proteins, essential nutrients don't get in from the gut to the bloodstream. Rather unhealthy proteins, polypeptides and toxins leak through the openings between the cells— the cell junctions.

Many natural enzymes can help digest proteins in the gut. The plant enzyme *bromelain* is derived from the pineapple plant. It can help digest proteins in the gastrointestinal tract—making up for a lack of protein-containing enzymes. An animal-derived pancreatic digestive enzyme is called *pancreatin*. It also digests protein that isn't properly digested by human pancreatic enzymes. These enzymes work as anti-inflammatory mediators and act like leukotrienes and prostaglandins in the normal human body.

Remember that herbal remedies must be anti-inflammatory, digestive in nature, mucilaginous, healing to the gut lining or antioxidant in nature. Typical herbal remedies include those containing the aloe vera extract, comfrey, licorice root, white willow bark, feverfew, devil's claw, yarrow, marshmallow and the yucca plant. We'll take a look at these herbal remedies more closely in a minute. Remember that, especially, if you're taking multiple herbal remedies, you'll need to see an herbalist who can recommend the best combination of herbs for your specific condition.

Fungicidal herbs include **garlic** and **Olive Leaf Extracts**. These are side effect-free and don't mix poorly with other herbal agents. Garlic contains potent antioxidants that help get rid of damaging oxygen free radicals that can damage DNA and cell membranes. It is useful in many diseases besides leaky gut syndrome, including heart disease and cancer. It also kills certain worms in the GI tract. Olive leaf extract is created from grinding olive leaves. It is believed to kill certain pathogens by inhibiting their replication process. It is used against viral infections and yeast infections of all types and can decrease their presence in the gastrointestinal tract.

Ginger is a good treatment for those who need anti-inflammatory strength as well as those who have nausea or motion sickness. The recommended anti-inflammatory dose is 1 to 2 grams of powdered ginger daily. Higher doses may be necessary for several months might be needed to get rid of the inflammatory process before going down to a lesser level.

Chaparral is also called creosote bush. It can be found in Southwestern United States and in Mexico as a weed that actually has serious antioxidant and anti-inflammatory properties. Medicinal chaparral is called Larrea tridentata and is used for many different diseases besides leaky gut syndrome, including tuberculosis, STDs, painful menstrual periods, snake bite and chicken pox. The US FDA warns against taking too much of the substance due to liver and kidney damage so you should definitely talk to an herbalist for proper dosing.

Prebiotics include fructo-oligosaccharides and inulin, which are digestible only to the friendly bacteria within the intestinal tract. They provide the "food" for the healthy bacteria to eat. They can be taken along with Lactobacillus acidophilus and Lactobacillus casei—healthy bacteria that use the food provided by the prebiotic agents.

Insoluble fiber comes from plants and helps clean out the gastrointestinal syndrome so that there isn't residual stool left in the colon, which is just fodder for bad bacteria to eat off of. Insoluble fiber can be taken in fiber bars, liquid emulsions of fiber or by eating fresh fruits and vegetables which contain insoluble fiber.

Barley grass supplement can be taken as a liquid or powder. Nutrients you can get from eating or drinking barley grass supplement include healthy amounts of beta carotene, calcium, potassium, manganese, Vitamin C, B vitamins, iron, phosphorus and copper. These are easily taken in by the body and absorbed for healthy nutrition.

Blue green algae can be very healthy for you and can contain healthy antioxidants protecting the gut from oxygen free radicals. Not all blue green algae are alike and some contain toxins. The kind you want to take in is called Aphanizomenon flos-aquae. It contains nearly all of the bioavailable vitamins you might need as well as Vitamin B12, carbohydrates that stimulate the migration of immune cells to the right place in the body, and essential fatty acids, such as DHA and omega-3 fatty acids.

Vitamin supplements will help create a healthy environment in which to heal from leaky gut syndrome. These include supplements containing, folate, magnesium, thiamine, zinc, vitamin B12, and biotin. If you can find a multivitamin that contains all of these elements, this would be perfectly good to take. Another healthy vitamin complex that works is high doses of B complex vitamins.

Marshmallow Root contains soothing agents that help the mucus membranes of the GI tract heal easily. Remedies out there that get rid of internal parasites that could be irritating the colon include red clover, wormwood, colloidal silver and garlic. Many of these need the advice and support of a good herbalist who can tell you how much you need to take to kill parasites in your body.

Licorice Root is good for leaky gut syndrome as well as its sequelae like various types of dermatitis and eczema. It has anti-allergic properties and anti-inflammatory properties.

Comfrey is an herb you'll want to take after talking with an herbalist because too much can cause liver problems. It contains a molecule called allantoin, which stimulates cell growth and repair in many body areas, including the gut. It is also an anti-inflammatory agent. Many take it topically for skin diseases related to leaky gut syndrome. Rashes of all types are helped through the use of topical comfrey. It also contains mucilage, saponins, pyrrolizidine alkaloids, inulin and healthy proteins. Many doctors and herbalists believe that comfrey should be reserved for its topical uses.

White Willow Bark, or Salix alba, is a natural fever and pain reducer that is good for those who have a fever or pain but don't want to take conventional anti-inflammatory agents that can be harsh on the gastrointestinal tract.

Feverfew, also called Tanacetum parthenium, is made from the crushed up leaves of the feverfew plant, which is a member of the sunflower family. It is a common folk remedy that is used for pain and fever in the place of harsh nonsteroidal anti-inflammatory medication. While it is commonly used for migraine headaches, it has good uses for all kinds of pain and fever in those who have leaky gut syndrome.

Yarrow is also called Achillea millefolium. Yarrow has anti-microbial properties and blood clotting properties. It is also well known for its anti-inflammatory properties and helps intestinal disorders as well as female reproductive tract inflammation. It can be used to treat early fever in patients who do not want to take nonsteroidal anti-inflammatory medications.

Yucca can be taken in capsule form. It is a potent anti-inflammatory medication that can be used to treat the inflammation of leaky gut syndrome. It has been used for many centuries by Native Americans and also seems to be helpful in treating joint inflammation and bleeding disorders.

Other herbal remedies for leaky gut syndrome include **Deglycyrrhizinated Licorice**, which is a seriously good anti-inflammation agent. It soothes the GI tract and helps those parts of the GI lining affected by aspirin and other nonsteroidal anti-inflammatory agents. Milk thistle can heal liver cells and protect it from toxic agents. It is also called silymarin. It increases the amount of healthy glutathione in the cells of the liver.

Aloe vera has natural healing powers so that it treats the damage to the lining of the GI tract. It contains mucilaginous polysaccharides that are anti-inflammatory in nature. All types of inflammation of the GI tract are helped by the addition of aloe vera. Aloe vera has antimicrobial properties and acts as an immune modulator.

Another herbal remedy is **slippery elm**. Slippery elm calms and soothes the damage in the lining of the gut. It has powerful antioxidant action which heals the lining of the GI tract. It also increases the amount of mucus in the GI tract, which has a protective effect on the mucosal lining. It is used for a number of external skin diseases and is taken internally to treat GI symptoms and respiratory symptoms. Leaky gut syndrome can be healed by slippery elm, which contains mucilage that is gel-like when mixed with water. It soothes the leaky gut with mucilage and protects the GI tract lining. Slippery elm also has many anti-oxidants in it that take care of GI inflammation. It stimulates the GI tract to make its own mucus secretion so the lining of the gut is further protected from food particles and pathogens.

Peppermint also soothes the gut and aids digestion when taken as an herbal supplement for leaky gut syndrome. Peppermint is good for things like headaches, anxiety, depression, nausea, diarrhea, flatulence and to kill bacteria, fungi, and viruses. It is a great herbal remedy for irritable bowel syndrome and indigestion.

You need to make sure that, for leaky gut syndrome and irritable bowel syndrome, you take enteric coated tablets that make it through the stomach and prevent heartburn that can occur if peppermint refluxes up the esophagus. Up to 80 percent of those who take peppermint for abdominal pain will get some relief.

Chamomile is an excellent choice of herbs for those with irritation, inflammation and problems with bacteria in the gut. It is taken orally as a capsule or in a tea. It helps people with sleep disorders, those with anxiety, wounds or burns, psoriasis, eczema and stomach problems. It has antispasmodic properties and reduces the inflammation in the stomach and intestines. Most people drink it as a tea twice a day because it tastes good and acts quickly to soothe the stomach.

Chamomile tea is a great home remedy for irritable colon or other irritations of the GI tract. Nausea is controlled and the amount of gas and bloating in the intestinal tract is reduced. Some side effects of taking chamomile include drowsiness and, in high doses, nausea, vomiting or skin reactions. The trick is to drink it or take it in using moderation. It is not recommended in pregnancy because it can cause miscarriages.

Echinacea is used for a number of illnesses and diseases and has been popular for hundreds of years. It appears to have some antimicrobial properties and is used for respiratory illnesses. Overall, Echinacea stimulates the immune system, reducing inflammation, killing viruses and having antioxidant properties.

It is used to treat infections of many kinds and to treat slow healing wounds. Because there are anti-inflammatory properties to Echinacea, it is good for an inflamed and leaky gut. Leaky gut has some infectious properties that are not healthy for the gut milieu. Those who have autoimmune diseases are helped by Echinacea, which helps the immune system be redirected toward fighting infection instead of fighting off normal body tissue. Just about any pathogen can be killed off by taking Echinacea.

Herbal remedies definitely have their place in the treatment and management of leaky gut syndrome. Once you know you have the diagnosis, sit down with a good herbalist who can take a look at the specific symptoms you have and can give you those that heal leaky gut syndrome. In addition, some of the herbal remedies aren't specific for leaky gut syndrome but provide pain or fever relief when non-steroidal anti-inflammatory medications are not indicated because of their negative effect on the gut.

Conclusion

Leaky gut syndrome can clearly happen to anyone but seems to be made worse by those who take antibiotics, those who take NSAIDS for pain and fever, and who are under a great deal of stress. Anything that changes the gut milieu so that good bacteria are killed off and bad bacteria take their place can result in leaky gut syndrome.

As you have learned, leaky gut syndrome happens when the physiology of the gut is changed so that the junctions between the cells that line the intestinal wall become greater because the cells themselves have shrunk. This allows molecules that are not "simple" molecules to pass into the bloodstream. These molecules can include polysaccharides (instead of simple sugars), polypeptides (instead of amino acids), complex fats (instead of fatty acids) and bacteria, viruses and bacterial particles.

These cause allergic reactions to occur to products that don't belong in the bloodstream.

Typically, this results in food allergies to food particles that have gotten through the cellular junctions and auto-immune reactions such as Crohn's disease, lupus and rheumatoid arthritis. These immune reactions are the result of foreign antigens that mimic antigens on the body's own tissue. Exactly what auto-immune disease comes out of getting leaky gut syndrome depends on which lookalike antigens are ingested by the body and which tissues they most resemble. Connective tissue antigens seem to be the most popular antigens created by leaky gut syndrome.

Some people with leaky gut syndrome have allergic symptoms like hives or urticaria. An itchy, bumpy rash can be the result of IgE mediated immune function. Other allergic symptoms like asthma and allergic nasal symptoms can also be caused by autoimmune antibodies or allergic reactions to substances a person ingests.

Both men and women can have estrogen dominance because ingested estrogen will enter the blood and take over those receptors responsive to estrogen. This can lead to premenstrual syndrome, uterine fibroids, breast tumors, breast cancer and uterine cancer. In men, it can lead to sexual dysfunction.

The liver becomes overwhelmed by the increase in toxic substances presented to it by the fact of having leaky gut syndrome. The toxins pass right through the overwhelmed liver and into the bile, where it is deposited into the small intestines and feeds back on itself to add even more toxins to the system. As you have read, there are many self-perpetuating aspects of leaky gut syndrome.

There are several modern tests for leaky gut syndrome, most of which test to see if large molecular weight molecules get into the bloodstream and urine after ingestion. They are good ways to see if the bowel is normal or if it has increased intracellular junctions.

Treating leaky gut syndrome depends on eating a healthy diet of foods that are soothing to the gut and that don't reduce the amount of acidity within the stomach—a necessary part of good digestion. Acidic foods seem to help and a diet that promotes healthy digestion can lessen the width of the leaky gut so that the process is stopped does a good job of taking care of the problem. Taking probiotics and prebiotics are also helpful in restoring the gut milieu so that healthy organisms predominate.

After you have identified the irritants responsible for leaky gut syndrome, such as alcohol, food allergies, NSAIDS and antibiotics, you need to follow a healthy diet. You also need to reduce stress as much as possible through the various stress reduction techniques.

Diet therapy may not rid the body of Candida or parasitic overgrowth. You may need to consider taking Nizoral or Diflucan, both antifungal agents that reduce fungal growth. If a stool sample shows you have worms, you can treat them with antihelminthic agents. Taking these medications may be harsh on your system so do so with the advice of an alternative medical specialist who can take care that you don't take the wrong medications at the wrong dose.

There are many nutritional supplements and herbal remedies useful for the various aspects of leaky gut syndrome. You need to consider seeing an herbalist who can recommend herbal remedies in the doses and types necessary to help your problem. Things like ginkgo, slippery elm, bioflavonoids, quercetin, chlorophyll complex and aloe vera are healthy herbal supplements you can choose from in order to treat leaky gut syndrome. Any supplement that has antioxidant properties can rid the body of oxygen free radicals and can improve health.

Interestingly, it is believed in traditional Chinese medicine that having leaky gut syndrome for a long time eventually leaches out Chi or Qi from your spleen, which is important in the management of your immune system. The damage to your liver and spleen do damage to the ability to absorb healthy food and your gut becomes leakier.

Living with leaky gut syndrome can be miserable but it is something you don't have to live with for the rest of your life. You can use the techniques as instructed in this manual and, before long, many of your symptoms will abate.

Made in the USA
Las Vegas, NV
05 March 2025

19113482R00074